EKG Interpretation Basics Guide:

Electrocardiogram Heart Rate Determination, Arrhythmia, Cardiac Dysrhythmia, Heart Block Causes, Symptoms, Identification and Medical Treatment Nursing Handbook

By

Brittany Samons

Table of Contents

Introduction

Chapter 1. Basic Principles of EKG (Electrocardiogram) Interpretation

Chapter 2. How Does The EKG Work?

Chapter 3. Cardiac Dysrhythmia

Chapter 4. Arrhythmia

   How to Identify Arrhythmia

   Arrhythmia Types

   Cardiac Arrhythmia Causes

   Symptoms of Arrhythmia

   Treatment For Cardiac Arrhythmia

   Heart block

Final Words

Thank You Page

EKG Interpretation Basics Guide: Electrocardiogram Heart Rate Determination, Arrhythmia, Cardiac Dysrhythmia, Heart Block Causes, Symptoms, Identification and Medical Treatment Nursing Handbook

By Brittany Samons

© Copyright 2015 Brittany Samons

Reproduction or translation of any part of this work beyond that permitted by section 107 or 108 of the 1976 United States Copyright Act without permission of the copyright owner is unlawful. Requests for permission or further information should be addressed to the author.

This publication is designed to provide accurate and authoritative information in regard to the subject matter covered. This work is sold with the understanding that the publisher is not engaged in rendering legal, accounting, or other professional services. If legal advice or other expert assistance is required, the services of a competent professional person should be sought.

First Published, 2015

Printed in the United States of America

Introduction

EKG interpretation is a clinical skill that is invaluable and many different ways are used to teach this in medical schools. The teaching method is at most times informal and they are expected to know how to do it while they are dealing with patients in the wards and clinics. In bookstores, you can easily purchase books that offer information, but most of their contents are too simple and detailed in a hopeless way. These books can be too complicated for some readers or incomplete and this book will make it simpler for you to better understand the interpretation basics of ECG.

You will find here the basic principles EKG, how it works, how you will be able to identify arrhythmia, heart attack, what causes them, what the symptoms are, and the medical treatments that are used today to treat these diseases. One by one each factors will be discuss help you understand how to apply them especially if you are interested in the field of medicine. It was written specifically for people who wish to understand more about EKG and give them a more in-depth look on how to interpret EKG results.

Heart diseases are responsible for the deaths of millions of lives in this world and it is important that people are informed about the symptoms, treatments, and what they can do to prevent it because it is always better. It is more convenient to work on prevention rather than having to deal with chronic heart diseases for the rest of your life. Being more aware of the threat it has to human life will make you think twice about your lifestyle habits, the food you eat, and where you are exposing yourself too. You should also become more aware if heart disease runs in the family because you have a higher chance of developing heart disease if you are not careful. Read this book so you will be enlightened more about the realities of heart diseases and how to interpret EKG results.

Chapter 1. Basic Principles of EKG (Electrocardiogram) Interpretation

In order to interpret the electrocardiogram findings, there are principles that need to be applied to avoid making mistakes when interpreting EKG results because it can be a matter of life and death. These principles were made to make it easier for people and especially the people in the medical field. There is usually no formal training as to how it should be interpreted because they are expected to learn it while they are dealing with a patient in the ward or in the hospital in general.

ECG GRID – This is seen as a voltage that is on a plot and the leads found on the vertical axis against the time seen on the axis that are horizontal are what they use to measure it. In order to detect the difference, in the galvanometer the electrodes are connected here. There is a pen on the ECG and it becomes deflected by a certain distance which would depend on the voltage that was measured.

Complexes and intervals – The electrocardiogram is normally composed of waveforms that differ which represents electrical details that happen during every cardiac cycle in all different parts of the heart. The waves used to label ECG are in alphabetical order starting from the P wave, then the QRS complex, and the S-T-T-U complex. The junction found at the end of the QRS complex and the start of the ST segment is called the J point.

P wave – This one stands for the right then the left atrial depolarization and it is low amplitude with a positive deflection which precedes the QRS complex. The general duration is 0.12 seconds and has an amount of 0.25 mv amplitude (2 ½ small boxes). Since the left atrium is preceded by the right atrial depolarization, the P wave is often seen notched in the leads of the limb which can be biphasic in lead V1. The deflection that is positive found in V1 is because of the right atrial depolarization that is anteriorly directed. You will also see that the second deflection that is negative stands for the left atrial depolarization that is posteriorly directed.

The depolarization of the atrial happens when the ventricular myocardium is also experiencing depolarization. So the "T wave" gets hidden by the QRS complex and it cannot be seen on the routine of the ECG. The PR interval becomes shorter when there is an increase in the heart rate. Repolarization of the atrial will be seen at the QRS' very end so the J point is altered. The J point will lower down and the ST segments will rapidly upslope which happens particularly during the first 80 msec which happens after the QRS complex has occurred. This change is normal and physiological, but it is essential that remembering when to interpret the ST segment that will change for ischemia.

PR interval – This interval is composed of both the P wave and the PR segment. It can be measured as soon as the P wave starts and up to the QRS complex's first part. It gives time for the atrial depolarization, AV node's conduction, and then through the His-Purkinje system's conduction. The heart rate changes the length of the PR interval, but normally the length is 0.14 to 0.20 sec. Faster heart rates make the PR interval shorter because of the AV nodal conduction's mediated enhancement. If the AV nodal conduction is slower, the rate becomes consequently longer leading to the tone to become sympathetic or it could be said as an increase in the vagal inputs.

QRS complex – This is the one that stands for the ventricular depolarization time. If the first deflection turns out to be negative, it is called the Q wave. You will often see q waves that are small in leads I, aVL, and V$ to V6. These are the result of a septal depolarization. If the first deflection is positive, this is called the R wave. This stands for the left ventricular system's depolarization. The depolarization of the right ventricular becomes obscured if the mass of the left ventricular myocardial is bigger than the right ventricle. The septal depolarization is represented by the wave lead found in V1. The deflection that is negative which follows the R wave is called the S wave. This stands for the high lateral wall's depolarization. In case there is a positive that comes second, it is called the 'R'. The small letters q,r, and s are used to represent the small amplitude waves that are less than 0.5 mV which means that it is 5 mm lesser than the standard calibration. A QRS complex that is entirely negative is known as the QS wave. The QRS is not influenced by the heart rate and it usually lasts for 0.6 to 0.10 seconds.

Observing the R wave progression that is on the precordial leads from VI to V6 is important. Usually an

R wave on the lead of V1 is seen that has an S wave that is deep. When it progresses to V6, the amplitude of the R wave will increase because of the increase of the left ventricular forces and this happens when there lesser deep waves. This is called R wave progression that is seen happening across the precordium.

ST Segment – This happens after the ventricular depolarization's ending even before the beginning of the repolarization. It happens when there is electrocardiographic silence. The first part of the ST segment is called the J point.

T wave – The T wave stands for the repolarization of the ventricular. Due to the slow rate of the repolarization compared to the depolarization, it will show an upstroke that is slow, and then it will rapidly return to its isoelectric line that can be seen following the peak. This means that both the amplitude and the asymmetric are both variable. The T should be seen going on a smooth movement of up and down. In case that the T wave appears to be irregular, considering a superimposed P wave is also good.

QT interval – This is composed of the QRS complex, which stands for the small part of the interval, and the segments of ST and T wave which both have a duration that are longer. This means that the QT interval is mainly used for measuring the repolarization of the membrane, but when it comes to clinical medicine, they also measure the QT interval. In case there is an increase in the QRS complex duration, this calls for a consideration that it should be measured. So any amount of the QRS complex that is seen becoming wide beyond 0.10 seconds, this should be lessened from the QT interval that is being measured.

U wave – This wave can be seen in other leads specifically the V2 to V4 leads. The uncertainty of the wave causes this, but it has been implied that it stands for the His-Purkinje system's depolarization that is known as the myocardium's repolarization. It can also stand for a mechanical event called the ventricular relaxation papillary muscle's repolarization. The U wave's amplitude is 0.2 mV less than it is evidently separated apart from the T wave. It becomes clearer in the event of hypokalemia. The U wave can have the tendency to merge if the QT interval has been prolonged, or it can become really obvious when there is a short ST interval.

Heart rate – If there is a regular cardia rhythm, the successes of the QRS complexes in between intervals will be seen basing from the grid of the ECG grid.

If there is a large box interval between 2 successes, it means that the heart is 300 beats per minutes. If there is an interval of 2 large boxes, it means that the heart rate is 150 beats per minute. Extrapolation can be performed in case the successes happen between the large boxes. Also, if the successive QRS complexes' interval falls between 1 and 2 boxes that are large, then the 5 small boxes 0.04 seconds stands for 30 beats per minute. If it falls between 2 to 3 boxes, the small boxes stand for 10 beats per minute. If it's between four to five boxes, it means that 5 beats per minute is represented by each box.

AXIS – This is electrical signal that is recorded on the ECG which has information that is relative to the magnitude and direction of complexes that very. The direction's average of the complexes can be identified.

Chapter 2. How Does The EKG Work?

The EKG machine is used to the transthoracic interpretation of the heart's electrical activity that occurs through time that has been captured and externally and skin electrodes were able to record it. The ECG device provides recoding that is noninvasive.

The ECG primarily aims to detect and amplify the small electrical shifts that happen when the depolarization of the heart muscle occurs in every heartbeat. When the heart is resting, there is an outer wall charge or cell membrane that occurs due to the heart's muscle cell. Depolarization is the term given to refer to the reduction of the charge towards zero. There is something inside the cell that is responsible for activating the mechanisms that causes it to contract. When each heart beat happens, if the heart is healthy, it will have a progression of the wave of depolarization that is orderly because it will be trigged by the cells present in the sinoatrial node, then it will go to the right atrium, then it will pass through the intrinsic pathways before being distributed to the ventricles. This will be seen by the very small rises and falls seen in the voltage located between electrodes is found at the side of the heart that is seen as the wavy line seen on the paper or screen. This will represent the overall rhythm of the heart that is weak in the different sections of the heart muscle.

Chapter 3. Cardiac Dysrhythmia

What is Cardiac dysrhythmia?

Cardiac dysrhythmia is when the person is having a heart beat that is not normal. The rhythm can have a pacing that is not regular or there is really low or high heart rate. There are types of dysrhythmia which can pose threat to a person's life, but there are types of dysrhythmias which are normal.

Sinus arrhythmia is a type of cardiac dysrhythmia that is considered normal.

What causes cardiac dysrhythmia

Inside and outside forces can lead to cardiac dysrhythmia. Outside forces include emotional stress, overexertion, exhaustion, drinking alcohol, and smoking. Taking in stimulants like decongestant, cocaine, and caffeine can also cause cardiac dysrhythmia. The inside forces that can cause cardiac dysrhythmia are thyroid problems, inflammatory diseases, automatic nervous system malfunction, and birth defects. The automatic nervous is responsible for carrying nerve impulses coming from the brain and also from the spinal cord towards the heart. The very main cause of serious cases of cardiac dysrhythmia is heart disease like abnormal heart valves, congenital heart disease, and coronary artery disease.

How to treat Cardiac dysrhythmia

Varying heart beats is normal, but there are some types of cardiac dysrhythmia which need medication or electric shock. Putting a battery powered pacemaker can also be a treatment because it sends electrical signals using an electrode that is placed near the heart's wall. A defibrillator is a device that is used to detect abnormal rhythm and brings one or more than one jolts of energy that will bring back the heart's normal rhythm. This can replace a blocked pathway or a pacemaker that is defective. A surgical technique called Catheter Ablation utilizes a very small device that is located at the end of the catheter which is a flexible tube that is brought inside the heart to remove the main cause of the abnormal rhythm by burning it away.

Chapter 4. Arrhythmia

How to Identify Arrhythmia

This is also known as the problems found in the rhythm of the heart and this happens when the electrical impulses that are responsible for coordinating your heart are not doing are not working properly. When you are experiencing this, your heart will start to beat fast, too slow or it becomes irregular. A person will feel as if there is a fluttering in the heart and their heart beat is rising. This is nothing to worry about, but sometimes arrhythmias can cause symptoms that ate life-threatening and could bother you.

If a person decides to get arrhythmia treatment, their heart beat can be controlled and fast and irregular heart beat can be eliminated. Sometimes, arrhythmias can worsen which is caused by a weak heart. You can reduce the risk of arrhythmia by having a healthy lifestyle.

Cardiac arrhythmia

Cardiac arrhythmia is a problem related to the heart rate's rhythm. When a person is experiencing cardiac arrhythmia, the heart beat can become irregular, too fast or too slow.

When a heart is beating too fast, it is called tachycardia. If the heart is beating too slow, it is called bradycardia.

Majority of the arrhythmias do not harm the body, but some cases can become life threatening or serious. When there is arrhythmia, the supply of blood in the body might not be enough because the heart cannot pump blood functionally. This can harm the organs, heart, and the brain.

Arrhythmia Types

Supraventricular arrhythmia- These are the arrhythmias that are occurring above the ventricle. "Supra" pertains to above and the ventricular refers to the ventricles.

Premature contractions – These are the heart beats that are considered extra and they come from the upper chamber of the heart (atrial).

Paroxysmal supraventricular tachycardia – This is a rhythm that is rapid or regular and it comes from above the ventricles.

Accessory pathway tachycardia – your heart beat will be on rapid stage because this is the result of an extra connection. The extra pathways are where the impulses will travel through and also the AV-His-Purkinje system. This will let the impulses to quickly travel the heart which will make the heart rate irregularly fast.

Reentrant tachycardia AV nodal– This is a fast heart rate that comes from the atria.

Atrial fibrillation – This is a very well-known irregularity in the heart's rhythm. A lot of the impulses will start to spread to the atria because it is fighting to travel through the AV node. The rhythm will become disorganized, irregular, and rapid. This is because of the impulses traveling in an orderly fashion through the atria. It can cause coordination to be lost and atrial contraction.

Atrial flutter – This is because of the rapid circuit that happens in the atrium. This is more regular and organized compared to atrial fibrillation.

Ventricular arrhythmias- These start from the lower heart chambers.

Premature ventricular contractions – These will begin in the heart's lower chambers and they are very early beats. This is very common and usually they do not give out any symptoms does not need any treatment. Sometimes, this is something that is related to stress, too much consumption of nicotine and caffeine. Those who are experiencing lots of PVCs should consult a doctor.

Ventricular tachycardia – This is a rhythm which comes from the heart's lower chambers. The rapid rate causes the heart from not being able to be filled sufficiently with blood which causes less blood to be pumped throughout the body. This could become a type of arrhythmia that is more serious especially for people who have heart disease. This can cause more symptoms and a heart doctor should take a look at this.

Ventricular fibrillation – This is an erratic and disorganized impulses that are being fired coming from the ventricles. This will cause the ventricles to start quivering and not be able to contract and pump blood throughout the entire body. This is considered to be a medical emergency and cardiopulmonary resuscitation together with defibrillation must be immediately performed.

Long QT syndrome – The interval area of the electrocardiogram is called the QT interval and this refers to the time it will take for the heart muscle to be able to contract and then recover and also firing of the electrical impulses and then to recharge. When this interval becomes longer than the usual, there will be an increased risk of having torsade de pointes which is a form of ventricular tachycardia that can become life-threatening.

Bradyarrhythmias- These are heart rhythms that are slow which can come from diseases found in the conduction system of the heart.

Sinus node dysfunction – This slow heart rhythm is caused by the abnormality in the sinus node.

Heart block – If there is a blockage in the electrical impulses of the heart when it goes through the sinus nodes going to the ventricles.

Cardiac Arrhythmia Causes

Below are the causes of cardiac arrhythmia:

- A thyroid gland that is overactive known as hyperthyroidism

- A heart attack that is happening at the moment

- A tissue has been scarred because of a heart attack that happened

- Smoking

- A thyroid gland that is underactive known as hypothyroidism

- Consuming too much caffeine or alcohol

- Stress

- Air pollution

- Some medications even under prescription

- Electric shock

- Change in the structure of the heart. One example of this is cardiomyopathy.

- Coronary artery diseases that is caused by blocked arteries

- High blood pressure

- Diabetes

Symptoms of Arrhythmia

Sinus node dysfunction usually has no symptoms, but it is the reason when a person feels fatigue and dizziness. Another one is the atrial fibrillation which will normally not show any symptoms, but it can cause a person to palpitate, faint, become weak, angina, and have a shortness of breath. If you feel chest pain, you should be aware that you are experiencing angina this is due to the very little blood supply that the heart is receiving.

When a person has atrial fibrillation, they can sometimes have an irregular heart beat or very normal heart beats. If a person has heart block, they are only experiencing fist degree if they are not seeing any symptoms. If irregular impulses start to occur, it means that they have a second degree heart block. Third degree heart block can cause a person to have a slow heartbeat, faint, and become dizzy. The VT will not show any symptoms or fluttering in the chest that is only mild. VT can cause a person to experience lightheadedness. This can cause a person to become unconscious or even cause death. Ventricular fibrillation can cause no pulse and can lead to death.

Treatment For Cardiac Arrhythmia

For people who have sinus node dysfunction, it is treated by putting a permanent pacemaker in the heart. Supraventricular tachyarrythmia treatment will entirely depend on what caused the arrhythmia. For some people, they can stop the problem by just applying massage to the carotid sinus found in the neck while some people would need to get medications such as beta-blockers, calcium channel blockers, lanoxin, digoxin, amiodarone, and cordarone. There are also some people who can respond to radiofrequency catheter ablation which is the only procedure that works for them. You will found a tissue in the AV-node that you should get rid of in order to prevent the exceeding electrical impulses from reaching the atria towards the ventricles. Atrial fibrillation is due to hyperthyroidism and to treat this you must undergo surgical process. Fibrillation is caused by rheumatic heart disease and this can be cured by heart valves being replaced. In order to lessen the heart rate, medications called beta-blockers, amiodarone, and digoxin should be taken. The amiodarone can be taken because it helps in reducing chances of atrial fibrillation to happen again. Catheter ablation, radiofrequency, and electrical cardioversion – a procedure done to bring a timed shock to the heart which aims to restore the heart's normal rhythm is an alternative treatment for atrial fibrillation.

Heart block

This is a problem with the electrical system of the heart which is responsible for controlling the heart rate and the heartbeat rhythm.

In every heartbeat there is an electrical signal spreading across the heart that are coming from the upper and lower chambers. When it is travelling, the signal makes the heart contract and pump blood.

There is a heart block if the electrical signal is slowed down or disrupted when it is moving inside the heart.

An AV-block is a type of heart block and if it's only first degree, does not need any treatment. Those who have second degree, frequent EKGs can be used to monitor this if they are not experiencing any symptoms and their heart rate is enough for them to perform activities daily. Some who have second degree heart blocks might need a pacemaker that is permanent. Those who have third degree heart blocks can be helped by a pacemaker. The ventricular tachycardia (VT) does not require any treatment if does not cause any damage that are structural to the heart if it is not a sustained one. If the person has a sustained VT, they will definitely need treatment. They can choose between an electromagnetic shock or intravenous medication which are both good for restoring the normal rhythm of the heart. The ventricular fibrillation is treated by sending electric shocks to the heart that are measured in order to restore the heat's normal rhythm. The electric shock is delivered to the heart during the occurrence of an emergency. Those who have gone through ventricular fibrillation, but have survived and those who have the risk of developing it, there is a high chance that they will be advised to have an implantable cardioverter defibrillator which is very similar to what is known as the pacemaker. This has wires that will be attached to the heart to connect a source of energy that is placed using surgery under the skin. This requires an operation.

Final Words

There are a lot of factors that can cause heart disease and it is really up to the individual to prevent the development of heart disease. This is one of the most causes of death in humans that are taking millions of lives today. You should always stay informed and aware if you are experiencing any of the said symptoms. Even if some of them are said to be harmless, it can still lead to more serious conditions and discomfort especially if you become dizzy or unconscious. Heart diseases can also be caused by complications of diabetes which is also a common disease among people today.

If you have diabetes, it does not mean that you will not have any heart disease. The heart disease that is gotten from diabetes is because of the complications that come with diabetes so you should also be careful. If you look at the causes of heart disease, they are mostly out of the habits that people have like drinking, smoking, getting no sleep, drugs, and taking dietary supplements. This is also a very noticeable cause of heart disease because they are the things that people are used to doing as part of their lives daily or occasionally. You might not see the complications of what you are doing now, but you will definitely experience the perils of your bad habits in the future. Anything in excess is bad and you must take proper responsibility for yourself and the people around you.

Other people may not have the privilege to know about the causes, symptoms, and treatments of heart diseases, but you do. By reading this book, you were given a brief information about the reality of heart disease so you must be able to share what you know to other people as well. Take the time to inform them what you have read in this book so that you will be able help other people and possibly alarm them in case they have been experiencing small symptoms, but are not aware of what can happen. The best thing to do is to consult your doctor in the event that you are experiencing symptoms because you deserve to know what is happening in your body. The heart needs to be treated well because it is responsible for everything that is functioning in the body. Without the heart, you will not have blood pumped all throughout the body which could mean that all of your organs will not work. If you are at the risk of developing heart disease, think about what you have been doing wrong and refine the way you live by getting proper diet and exercise. Without proper diet, you will not be able to function well even when you are exercising. You will feel that your energy level is down when you are exercising because your diet is not good.

The number one thing you should remember to do is to take care of yourself because you deserve good health and the people around you need to be influenced by you. If you are smart to take care of yourself this only means that you can contribute something to the world. Do not be influenced by other people's bad habits because it will only cause you to have health problems.

Now, change the way you live and be the best version of yourself.

Thank You Page

I want to personally thank you for reading my book. I hope you found information in this book useful and I would be very grateful if you could leave your honest review about this book. I certainly want to thank you in advance for doing this.

If you have the time, you can check my other books too.

www.ingramcontent.com/pod-product-compliance
Lightning Source LLC
LaVergne TN
LVHW021744060526
838200LV00052B/3469